ENERGY POWERHOUSE

A major form of energy storage, creatine powers muscle contraction for bursts of activity. Scientific research has verified that creatine increases muscle strength, lean body mass and muscle energy while accelerating energy recovery during intense exercise. World-class athletes have the competitive advantage that comes from correct use of this natural fuel. Dr. Richard Passwater and sports medicine experts tell you how to use creatine to enhance your athletic performance safely and effectively.

ABOUT THE AUTHOR

Richard A. Passwater, Ph.D. is one of the most called-upon authorities in preventive health care. A noted biochemist, he is credited with popularizing the term "supernutrition" in such books as *Supernutrition: Megavitamin Revolution* and *The New Supernutrition*. His many other works include *Cancer Prevention and Nutritional Therapies* and *Pycnogenol*. Dr. Passwater lives in Berlin, Maryland, where he is the director of a research laboratory.

Creatine

Enhancing muscular functioning, this safe, natural dietary supplement helps athletes achieve better performance and strength quickly

Richard A. Passwater, Ph.D.

Keats Publishing, Inc. ⚹ New Canaan, Connecticut

ACKNOWLEDGMENTS

I enjoyed the opportunity to write this book about creatine and hope that it will help many achieve their goals and dreams. The task was made easy thanks to the generous help of Anthony Almada, Paul Greenhaff, Ph.D., Brett Hall, Bill Phillips and Mike Prevost, Ph.D.

Creatine is intended solely for informational and educational purposes and not as medical advice. Please consult a medical or health professional if you have questions about your health.

Keats Good Health Guides are published by
Keats Publishing, Inc.
27 Pine Street (Box 876)
New Canaan, Connecticut 06840

Keats Publishing website address: www.keats.com

Contents

INTRODUCTION

There has been a great deal of excitement among athletes about the dietary supplement creatine. Scientific research has verified that creatine is not just an energy source that powers muscles–it is much more. Creatine is becoming the athlete's most important supplement because it:

• Increases muscle strength

• Promotes significant increases in muscle size (lean body mass) without increases in body fat or water content

• Increases muscle energy (more energy available per unit time) and improves performance during short-duration "bursts," high-intensity and intermittent exercise or activity

• Accelerates energy recovery between bouts of intense exercise (for example, after a sprint, the next sprint would be easier and at greater speed than without creatine)

• May reduce fatigue by reducing lactic acid build-up in short-burst exercises, and

• Permits more intense training which further improves strength and muscle growth by delaying muscle fatigue. (Creatine regenerates ATP-energy to increase muscle-working time in anaerobic activity such as training to failure)

These are not claims, but facts proven by extensive scientific study by experts at leading university and sports medicine research centers around the world. You will hear from some of these experts in this book.

In addition to the above proven benefits, there are several more possible benefits of creatine that have not been proven in humans, but suggestions from animal studies or test-tube type studies are strong enough to warrant further research. These include:

• Promotion of muscle growth (muscle protein synthesis, muscle

fiber size and muscle cell volume) which has been shown in the case of creatine-deficient humans having gyrate atrophy
• Helps in sparing muscle fibers from degradation (more work with less catabolism)

In addition to the above benefits, some claims have been made for creatine that are definitely incorrect. Creatine does **not** increase aerobic endurance.

World-class athletes have been following creatine research very closely as most have found significant increases in performance with this ergogenic aid (work productivity enhancer). Creatine-trained athletes now dominate all aspects of track and field and swimming.

The story of this book begins with a seminal conference held in Bethesda Maryland, June 3 and 4, 1996. I mention that because it is a day that I will never forget! Why? Because our highest government scientific institutes were sponsoring the presentation of good scientific evidence that dietary supplements can help normal, healthy, well-nourished, active people improve their performance. The conference was a National Institutes of Health (NIH) workshop entitled "The role of dietary supplements for physically active people," and was cosponsored by eleven divisions of the NIH.

The National Institutes of Health had invited Dr. Paul Greenhaff from the University of Nottingham in England to brief the newly formed NIH Office of Dietary Supplements. His topic was "Does dietary creatine supplementation have a role to play in exercise metabolism?" British and Swedish researchers had been publishing their scientific studies on the benefits of creatine in athletic performance, and athletes had taken notice.

The discovery of the benefits of creatine loading by the Swedish researchers Drs. Eric Hultman, Roger Harris and Karin Soderlund of the Karolinska Institute in Sweden parallels the discovery of the benefits of carbohydrate loading, also by Dr. Hultman and his colleagues in the 1960s. However, while "carbo-loading" increases performance by increasing the amount of carbohydrate fuel (glycogen) stored in muscles, creatine loading increases the energy stored in muscles plus helps muscles grow bigger and stronger.

Dr. Greenhaff later collaborated with Dr. Hultman to refine the concept of creatine loading and maintenance to enhance sports performance. These studies were published in 1993 and 1994. Dr. Greenhaff will discuss these concepts clearly and simply later in this book.

Articles in athletic magazines occasionally mention a rumor that

USSR and Bulgarian athletes may have been using creatine for many years, perhaps since the 1970s, to power their Olympic athletes. Neither I, nor those in the creatine field of research with whom I have discussed this, however, have found any scientific documentation of this use. A few former Soviet athletes may have mentioned that they were fed creatine phosphate or were given creatine phosphate injections. While this may be true, it is apparent that whatever the form of the creatine and its dosage, this may not be the same as the creatine loading and saturation concepts being used today by world-class athletes.

It appears that the first documented use of creatine supplementation was with the British athletes training for the 1992 Olympics in Barcelona. Creatine was credited with powering several of the British athletes to gold medals. *The London Times* (August 7, 1992) reported that Linford Christie, the 100-meter gold medalist, trained with creatine before the 1992 Olympics; and *Bodybuilding Monthly* reported that Sally Gunnell, the 400-meter gold medalist, also trained with creatine. *The London Times* also reported that Colin Jackson, the champion British 110-meter hurdler, just began taking creatine right before the Olympics. Although he did not win the gold medal at the Olympics, he soon beat the Olympic gold medalist, Mark McCoy, on several occasions.

Shortly thereafter, U. S. champion athletes began using creatine. Since then, scientists have elucidated more "secrets" on how best to utilize creatine for optimal benefit. Now champion athletes from most countries are using creatine supplements. The list of U. S. athletes is a "Who's Who" in track and field. Three out of four medal winners are using creatine, and the rest will probably follow suit once they discover this "competitive edge." **The point is that it will be difficult for those who don't properly use creatine supplements to compete against creatine-trained athletes.**

Low-potency creatine supplements were originally available in Britain, but creatine supplements especially designed for performance and strength enhancement were not commercially available until about 1993. In 1993, researchers Anthony Almada, B.Sc., M.Sc. and Edward Byrd introduced their formulation based on reports in the scientific literature, plus their own research. In late 1992 and early 1993, the results seemed so unbelievable that they had little success convincing established companies to introduce creatine supplements in a convenient form athletes could use to achieve creatine loading and maintenance. Thus they formed their own company, which became incorporated in mid-1993, and introduced the first commercial product especially designed to take advantage of their scientific research. Since that time, nearly all of the companies making sports nutrition supplements have introduced kindred products.

Judging from the 50,000+ hits on creatine Internet web pages in just a few months' time and the expanding pages of creatine advertisements in body-building magazines, the secret is out. However, the various ads and web pages can be confusing to the reader. The very day that I started writing this book, I received a telephone call from a reporter for the Pennsylvania State University newspaper asking for clarification of a few technical points about creatine supplementation. Even though Pennsylvania State University had reported about creatine supplementation in the *Penn State Sports Medicine Newsletter* (Vol. 2, No. 5, January 1994), the reporter still found the claims and counterclaims confusing. The goal of this book is to simplify the science of creatine supplementation, separate fact from theory and misinformation and present a practical guide to the safe and efficacious use of creatine to help you achieve your goals.

After studying 200 articles in the applicable scientific literature on creatine and muscle function (see bibliography for some of these) and interviewing some of the primary researchers and manufacturers, the creatine timeline seems to be as follows. Creatine was discovered in meat extracts in 1832 by the French scientist Michel-Eugene Chevreul, who named it after the Greek word for flesh. By 1923, it was known that the average human body contained over 100 grams of creatine stored in muscle tissue. In 1981 there was an article in the *New England Journal of Medicine* by Dr. I. Sipila and colleagues that reported that supplementation with 1.5 grams of creatine in a group of patients having gyrate atrophy led to greater strength. The creatine supplement increased body weight by 10 percent after one year and partially reversed the type II muscle fiber atrophy associated with this disease. Type II muscle is "fast" muscle tissue. One athlete in the group improved his record for the 100-meter sprint by two seconds.

In the late 1980s, Dr. Eric Hultman and his colleagues discovered the concept of creatine loading. Perhaps due to the importance of this new concept and the need for thorough peer-review, publication in the scientific literature did not occur until 1992. In 1993, Dr. Paul Greenhaff and his colleagues were the first to show creatine's beneficial effects on intense exercise. In 1994, Anthony Almada, Conrad Earnest and their colleagues presented their data showing the ability of creatine to increase strength during weightlifting (bench press) and the finding that weight gain associated with creatine use was due to increases in muscle (lean body mass). These results were published in 1995.

Creatine is a major form of energy storage used to power muscle contractions for bursts of activity. Supplementation of the diet with generous amounts of creatine can improve the performance of every type of athlete–power athletes and speed athletes alike, whether male or female. Champion sprinters, swimmers, distance runners, cyclists, weight lifters, bodybuilders, skiers, wrestlers, boxers and team sport athletes use creatine. The advantages that creatine gives most of them is enormous. I say "most" because like all else involving humans, everything doesn't work for everybody all the time. Research shows that creatine helps 80 percent or more of those who use it correctly. This percentage should increase even more with newer methods of creatine use discussed in this book.

Creatine is a compound naturally made in our bodies to supply energy to our muscles. Its chemical name is methyl guanidine-acetic acid. The structure of creatine is

$$NH2 - C (NH) - NCH2(COOH) - CH3$$

N=Nitrogen   C=Carbon   O=Oxygen   H=Hydrogen

CREATINE IS MADE IN OUR BODIES

Virtually all (95 to 98 percent) of the body's creatine is stored in skeletal muscles, with the remainder found in heart, brain and testes. An average-sized healthy male may have about 4 ounces (120 grams) of creatine stored in his body. When creatine is used up during work or exercise, the body normally makes another 2 grams a day as a replenishment. Muscles have two sources of supply for creatine. One source is the creatine made within the body, the other is the creatine supplied by the diet. Animal studies show that the liver, pancreas and kidneys produce creatine which is transported in the blood to the muscles. In humans, the liver is the major site of creatine biosynthesis, although some creatine may be made in the pancreas and kidneys. These organs can combine the amino acids arginine, methionine and glycine to form creatine.

Arginine + glycine→guanidinoacetic acid

Guadinoacetic acid + methyl group (CH3) from methionine→creatine

I will describe this process in a little more detail, as some manufacturers of creatine supplements are claiming that one product or another possibly stimulates creatine biosynthesis as well as supplies creatine itself. They refer to the precursor compounds as if everyone should know them by the three-letter acronyms. Whether or not these claims are accurate awaits clinical studies.

In the first step of creatine biosynthesis, a portion of the amino acid arginine is removed and added to the amino acid glycine to form a new compound called guanidinoacetic acid (GAA). The portion removed from arginine and transferred to glycine is a called an amidine group, and its transfer is made possible by the enzyme glycine transamidinase. It is correct to say that GAA is a precursor of creatine.

The second step involves removing a portion of a sulfur-containing compound called S-adenosylmethionine (SAM). SAM is derived from the amino acid methionine, so in essence, it can be said that creatine is formed from parts of three amino acids–arginine, glycine and methionine–and thus it is also correct to say that they are precursors of creatine. The portion transferred from SAM is called a methyl group, and its transfer to GAA is made possible by the enzyme guanidinoacetate methyltransferase. After the methyl group has been added to GAA, the resulting compound is called methyl guanidineacetic acid, or simply creatine.

In man, creatine is known to be made in the liver and, according to animal studies, is likely to also be made in the pancreas and kidneys; it is transported via the blood and taken up by muscle cells. Creatine is then converted into creatine phosphate (CP), also called phosphocreatine, by the enzyme creatine kinase (found inside muscle cells) through the addition of a high-energy phosphate group added. The bond in CP between an atom of phosphorus (P) on the phosphate group and an oxygen atom on creatine contains stored energy. When this bond is broken during a chemical reaction, energy is released. The cycling back and forth of creatine to creatine phosphate and back to creatine, etc., is very important to the process of supplying energy to muscle cells. We will discuss this in more detail later.

Some creatine, an average of about 2 grams per day depending on the muscle mass of the individual–the same amount that is normally biosynthesized–is lost from the body during this cycling process. This creatine forms creatinine which is then removed from the blood via the kidneys and excreted in the urine. Urine concentration of creatinine averages about one-tenth that of urea.

DIETARY SOURCES OF CREATINE

The richest food source of creatine is animal muscle such as that found in meats and fish. To increase sports performance, creatine supplements are usually taken in 5 gram doses, one to four times a day, depending on whether the athlete is in the loading phase or the maintenance phase. To obtain 5 grams of creatine from steak would require about 2.4 pounds (1.1 kilograms) of fresh, uncooked steak. Vegetarians have little creatine in their diets. Table 1 lists some dietary sources of creatine.

Table 1. Creatine in selected food items.

FOOD	AMOUNT of CREATINE (grams/pound)
Beef	2.0
Cod	1.4
Cranberries	0.009
Herring	3.0
Milk	0.05
Pork	2.3
Salmon	2.0
Tuna	1.8

Adapted from Balsom et al. *Sports Med.* 18(4):270 (1994)

THE BASICS OF MUSCLE FUNCTION

As Dr. John Fuller Jr. and I reviewed in our book on HMB (Keats Publishing, Inc., 1997), the body's more than 400 muscles contain about 250 million muscle cells. Muscles are tissues composed of fibers that are able to contract to move parts and organs of the body. Generally, muscles are classified into two types, smooth muscles and striated muscles. Striated muscles include the heart and skeletal muscles. Except for the heart, we can voluntarily control their movement. The heart is sometimes classified as a third type, but it is basically a striated muscle having slightly different responses to stimuli. Smooth muscles are muscles within hollow organs such as the stomach and intestines. About 40 percent of the average body is skeletal muscle, and perhaps another 10 percent is smooth and heart muscle. Of course, advanced body builders have a larger percentage of striated muscle in their bodies.

Muscles come in many sizes. The largest muscle is the quadriceps in the thigh, and the smallest is the stapedius muscle of the middle ear. The typical quadriceps muscle is a half-million times the size of the stapedius, which is only a few millimeters in length and a millimeter or two in diameter.

If you are interested in muscle fiber structure and the chemistry of muscle movement or growth, you may wish the visit "Introduction to Muscle" on the web site maintained by the University of California at San Diego. The URL or web address is http://muscle.ucsd.edu/mus-intro/over.html.

BUILDING MUSCLE MASS

As Dr. John Fuller Jr. and I also discussed in our booklet *Building Muscle Mass, Performance and Health With HMB* (Keats Publishing,Inc., 1997), muscle growth and size are related to the amount of use they receive. HMB is beta-hydroxy-beta-methylbutyrate, a dietary supplement that aids muscle growth. Nature is very conservative, and if something is not used it will be done away with. Nature's rule is, "use it or lose it." Nature sees no sense in having to feed big muscles if they aren't going to be used for anything. So if we don't use our muscles for hard work or exercise, they will atrophy to the size and strength needed for the amount of work to which they are subjected. At this point, the muscles will reach a steady state of no growth or atrophy where synthesis and breakdown are equally balanced. During muscle growth (in response to stimuli such as weight lifting) protein synthesis is greater than protein breakdown.

Additionally, muscles are continually using this balance of synthesis and breakdown to undergo a remodeling in the body. This means that muscle proteins are continually being replaced, sometimes in as little as a few weeks. During this remodeling, muscles can alter their diameters, lengths, strengths, neural (nerve) and blood supplies, energy-producing enzymes and even their type of muscle fiber. Again, muscles are affected by the amount of exercise or work performed. If they aren't exercised or worked, they will slowly atrophy, but with strenuous work the muscles will adjust by growing. That is, unless they are overworked, which could result in tearing down more muscle than can be built in a short time. So the important message is that muscle size is basically a function of the amount of work a muscle is asked to perform and that both catabolism and anabolism are important in determining how large a muscle will grow.

Many people have been taught that exercise builds muscles by first destroying the old muscle cells (catabolism) which are then replaced by new and stronger muscle cells (anabolism). This old paradigm is not accurate. Let's look at what has to occur to build muscle and strength.

Muscle growth is **not** a process of dying cells being replaced with new muscle cells. We pretty much have the same number of muscle fibers that we are born with throughout life. The process of building new muscle actually involves adding new nuclei and more protein within those fibers through a process called "hypertrophy." Each muscle fiber contains several hundred to several thousand myofibrils (slender strands). In turn, each myofibril contains about 1,500 myosin *filaments* and 3,000 actin filaments. The addition of nuclei and protein increase the number of actin and myosin filaments in each fiber, thus causing enlargement of these same muscle fibers. The greater number of actin and myosin filaments in the myofibrils (muscle fibers) induce these myofibrils to split within each muscle fiber to form new myofibrils.

Therefore, the process of building up muscle is the result of making new muscle protein and this, of course, is a fine balance between making protein (protein synthesis), and the normal process of tearing down proteins (proteolysis). Intense muscle exercise actually increases both protein synthesis and protein breakdown.

Muscle growth results from four factors working together:
- A stimulus that causes a contraction at or near maximal force
- Adequate energy present to power the contraction
- Adequate nutrients present to use in the building process. These nutrients include the amino acids used to form muscle protein and the vitamins and minerals used in the building of muscle proteins
- An adequate supply of all the materials needed to make the muscle cells grow. These include the nutrients that we eat, and compounds made from other materials within the muscle cells, as well as hormones and growth factors released by other body components

We still don't understand the complete story about how maximal muscle contraction leads to increased muscle growth, but studies show that creatine can help by providing the energy to contract our muscles harder and more frequently. Creatine also is believed to cause "cell volumizing," which appears to be a stimulus for muscle growth. This will be discussed later.

POWERING MUSCLES

The Energizer bunny will stop when his stored energy is depleted. The same is true with muscles. Muscles cannot generate energy from stored fuels fast enough so they rely on stored energy to make up the difference. The creatine phosphate (CP) made from creatine in muscles provides chemical energy from its high-energy phosphate group to immediately energize muscles on demand.

Energy Fuels

The body uses three main energy systems; two are anaerobic (oxygen-independent) and the third is aerobic (oxygen-dependent). One anaerobic system uses creatine and the other uses glycogen. The aerobic system uses a complicated cycle of biochemical reactions called the Krebs cycle (also called the citric acid cycle).

The creatine-based anaerobic system is the muscle's source of immediate energy and provides a very brief burst of energy. This system is called the "phosphagen system" (also called the "ATP-CP system" or "direct phosphorylation system"). In the phosphagen system, creatine phosphate (CP) (also called phosphocreatine) regenerates spent adenosine triphosphate (ATP). Working muscles need several hundred times as much ATP as those same muscles do when they are at rest. The phosphagen system provides immediate energy and the burst normally lasts for about 30 seconds, but with creatine loading, this time can be extended significantly. The purpose of this stored energy system is to provide the energy for immediate muscle contraction. The other energy systems cannot provide immediate energy, but they can kick in at later stages after the motion is started.

Dr. Greenhaff stated during his NIH lecture that the availability of CP is the most likely limitation to muscle performance during intense, fatiguing, short-lasting exercise, that is, where the anaerobic ATP demand is very high. His 1991 study implicated the availability of CP specifically in type II muscle fibers as being of critical importance to the maintenance of performance during maximal short-lasting exercise. Of course, the amount of free creatine in the muscle determines the amount of CP present.

Glycogen is the fuel for producing energy in the second anaerobic system used to power medium-duration activities. This energy system is called the anaerobic glycolysis system. Long-duration activities require activating the aerobic energy system which uses both glycogen and fats as fuel.

Long-duration activities use up many calories of energy. The body stores the calories for long-term activities in muscles as glycogen and as fat, which is more compact and calorie-dense. If an activity were to require 3,500 calories, the calories can be stored as 2.25 pounds of carbohydrate (glycogen or glucose) or 1 pound of fat. (These figures include associated water and proteins in the body tissue weight.)

As the body expends its ready reserves of carbohydrates, it shifts over to burning fat. This is achieved by enzymatically breaking down stored fats into free fatty acids. The free fatty acids are then converted into acetyl-CoA and other compounds and are carried through the Krebs cycle which produces ATP. The energy is efficiently stored as fat, but some energy and time are required to get this energy out of fat storage and back into a useable fuel to support muscle work.

Getting the Energy out of the Fuels

Energy is a force, not a compound. Energy can be stored in many ways such as the potential energy in an object that has been raised to a higher level and is at rest, or stored in a chemical compound by moving electrons into higher orbitals. ATP is the prime energy-containing molecule in the body and is used in thousands of biochemical reactions throughout the body.

We can account for the energy transferred in the body by keeping track of the formation and conversion of ATP. Biochemists like to think of ATP as acting as the "energy currency" of the cell. ATP is the currency used to transfer free energy derived from compounds of higher energy potential to those of lower energy potential.

ATP is formed via a cycle of reactions called the Krebs cycle. The calories of energy stored in food can be converted into ATP. The carbohydrates, fats and proteins in food can be broken down into smaller compounds. These smaller compounds, such as simple sugars and fatty acids, can be metabolized to pyruvic acid, which can enter the Krebs cycle. The aerobic pathway to forming ATP occurs in the mitochondria (the energy factory of a cell). The Krebs cycle combines the metabolized food products with oxygen and generates ATP in a process called oxidative phosphorylation.

That is more than an athlete really needs to know about using creatine supplements to increase athletic performance. However, today many athletes are becoming serious students of exercise physiology and biochemistry. If you have greater interest in understanding how creatine becomes locked into muscles to produce more energy, the Technical Box provides a more exacting description. If you are not interested in the biochemical details, please feel free to skip the Technical Box or even skip further ahead to the section on creatine loading, which is the most critical aspect in using creatine supplements to increase athletic performance.

Technical Box. Additional Details of Creatine Biochemistry

In muscle cells, glucose (blood sugar) enters the cytoplasm of the cell and is locked there by phosphorylation similar to the way creatine can be locked into muscle cells. The glucose is then converted to fructose and then to glyceraldehyde phosphates (GP). The cell can convert GP into pyruvate, which then enters the Krebs cycle and leads to the production of ATP. For each molecule of glucose that enters the muscle cell, theoretically, 36 molecules of ATP can be generated.

ATP production via the Krebs cycle is a relatively slow process. It takes a little priming to get the cycle revved up and it doesn't produce ATP fast enough for immediate response. The body needs immediate energy to fill in the period before aerobic, Krebs cycle-generated ATP kicks in. This source of ATP is obtained anaerobically from CP donating P to ADP.

The first energy to power muscles comes from stored ATP and CP. Then the body can shift into second gear by activating the anaerobic glycolysis system to use the fuel stored as glycogen in the muscle. The muscle cells break glycogen into glucose and eventually into pyruvate as described above. The pyruvate then enters the Krebs cycle to produce more ATP. Where do fats fit into the energy picture?

As the muscles are worked, they expend their supply of stored carbohydrates. During this process, some of the energy is converted into heat energy and the muscles warm up. The rise in temperature activates fat-burning enzymes, and the muscles shift into "third gear" by calling upon the calories stored as fats. This warm-up process takes time. As mentioned earlier, fat molecules consist of three fatty acids linked to a compound called glycerol, which has three carbon atoms and serves as the backbone of the fat molecule. When the body needs this extra energy stored in fat, it releases fat molecules from fat cells (some coming from fat stored in muscle cells) and breaks them back down into free fatty acids and glycerol.

A trained athlete can do this very efficiently because the required enzymes are readily available. Since Nature doesn't waste resources by making compounds that the body isn't using on a regular basis, a sedentary person doesn't have these necessary enzymes readily available in sufficient quantities. Thus, a sedentary person cannot reach back for this extra fuel to keep the muscles powered. A sedentary person will soon run out of gas because he can't burn fat efficiently and can't deliver oxygen to the cells fast enough. Training

Additional Details of Creatine Biochemistry (contd.)

not only strengthens the muscles and improves the nerve-muscle linkage, but also increases the amount of carbohydrate fuel stored in muscles,
improves oxygen efficiency and also increases the amount of enzymes available to convert fat into energy.

Other enzymes in muscle cells cleave portions of the fatty acids two carbon atoms at a time. The two-carbon fragments are converted into a compound called acetyl CoA, which can then enter the Krebs cycle (see glossary). For every two carbons in a free fatty acid (there are 18 -20 carbons typically in dietary fatty acids), theoretically 17 molecules of ATP can be formed (provided enough oxygen can be delivered to the cell).

The energy stored in ATP is released when a phosphate group is removed. ATP has a row of three phosphate groups attached to a larger adenosine group.

ATP: Adenosine - P~P~P (triphosphate)
ADP: Adenosine - P~P (diphosphate)
AMP: Adenosine - P (monophosphate)

When one of the phosphate groups is removed from ATP during a reaction, the energy that was stored in the bonds holding the outer-most phosphate group to middle phosphate group is also released (7.3 kcal/mole). This energy is the result of the charge repulsion of the adjacent negatively charged oxygen atoms in the phosphate group. ATP contains two high-energy phosphate groups (plus a "normal" phosphate group) and ADP contains both one high-energy phos-phate group plus a normal phosphate group.

The three phosphate groups in ATP are stabilized by the electric charge of magnesium ions. Magnesium, thus, is a mineral that is crit-ical to the energy process.

ATP does not act alone when it releases its high-energy phosphate group. This reaction is always coupled with another reaction and thus drives the reaction which wouldn't ordinarily be able to proceed by adding 30.5 kJ/mole of energy.

When ATP releases a phosphate, the molecule is left with two phos-phate groups, and the resulting compound is called, not surprisingly, adenosine diphosphate (ADP). The same series of reactions produces energy when ADP loses a phosphate and is converted to adenosine monophosphate (AMP). The high-energy phosphate group (P) that is released does not exist as a free phosphate, but is immediately

Additional Details of Creatine Biochemistry (contd.)

transferred to another compound such as creatine.

Creatine (C) enters the picture as creatine phosphate (CP). Most of the creatine that is taken up by muscle is converted into CP with the aid of an enzyme called creatine kinase (CK). Dr. Greenhaff has found that at rest, about two-thirds of the creatine in muscle is in the form of CP. The phosphate group comes from the phosphate groups previously cleaved from ATP and ADP. Thus, the phosphate is recycled back into ADP and ATP, and this biochemical reaction also adds energy to the molecules as the new phosphate bonds are formed. In the process, plain creatine is released from the CP. Now the cycle is ready to repeat again. All of this may sound technical, but the take-home message is that creatine, in the form of CP, refuels the energy compound ATP. Perhaps it will seem clearer when looked at in the chemist's shorthand shown below:

$$C + P = CP \text{ (with the help of creatine kinase)}$$
$$CP + ADP + H^+ = ATP + C$$

The H^+ in the second reaction is called a "hydrogen ion." This represents acid and points to the possibility of CP utilization during exercise to remove acid (lactic acid) that can accumulate. This point will be discussed later.

The more creatine stored in muscles, the more energy is available to activate the muscle. During intense work, the muscles may quickly be depleted of their creatine supply. If more creatine can be stored in the muscle, then more work can be done with greater intensity. Dietary supplementation can be used to load muscles with extra creatine.

CREATINE LOADING

Creatine loading is a method for maximizing the amount of creatine stored in muscles. As mentioned earlier, this concept was pioneered by Drs. Eric Hultman, Roger Harris and Karin Soderlund in 1992. Dr. Paul Greenhaff and his colleagues at the University of Nottingham worked with the Swedish group to help refine the concept of creatine loading and maintenance. Dr. Greenhaff will summarize his research for us, but first, let's look at how creatine gets into muscles.

When the amount of creatine stored in muscles is low, creatine is carried into muscle cells via a "sodium pump" (a common method the body uses to transport chemicals against a concentration gradient). As the amount of creatine in the muscle cells increases, this pump may be shut down, but if the amount of creatine in the blood is increased, then diffusion can push more creatine in. (The energy to overcome the concentration gradient probably comes from an energy-driven transporter protein on muscle cell membranes that is activated by guanidino groups.)

Another reason why the concentration of creatine in muscles can continue to increase is that once creatine gets into muscle cells, it can be converted into creatine phosphate (CP), which is trapped in the cells. Another lesser reason is that some creatine binds to components inside the cells.

The scientific studies have not examined the question of dosage: how much creatine to take per unit of body weight. The working hypothesis is that the objective is to saturate the creatine transport proteins with as much creatine as possible so that the muscles cannot take up any more. This is primarily a factor of transport capacity and not particularly a factor of body weight.

Let's look at what Dr. Greenhaff and his colleagues have learned. Dr. Greenhaff was kind enough to explain his research here expressly for your benefit.

Passwater: What is creatine loading?

Greenhaff: Creatine loading, as the wording implies, is a mechanism of increasing the creatine store of skeletal muscle, which in most people is in the region of 125 millimoles per kilogram of dry muscle (or about 16 milligrams per kilogram). By ingesting creatine in particular quantities you can increase the muscle creatine uptake by about 25 percent on average, but I should point out that the variation between individuals is quite large. This is a point which people seem to ignore at the moment. You do find individuals who actually don't respond to creatine ingestion.

Passwater: We'll pick up on that point shortly, but first, please tell us what is happening biochemically to achieve creatine loading?

Greenhaff: The mechanism of creatine transport into muscle is not completely resolved. There are several postulated methods of transport into muscle, but what is clear is, once creatine is in the muscle it is trapped there. Creatine doesn't leave the muscle at a very rapid rate, so once you have achieved creatine uptake, your stores remain elevated for quite some time, perhaps having a four-to-six week half-life. They are not degraded during exercise.

Passwater: How can creatine loading be achieved by athletes?

Greenhaff: Our studies show that probably the most effective way to creatine-load skeletal muscle is to ingest 20 grams of creatine for five days in four 5-gram doses each day and to ingest that with a simple-sugar carbohydrate solution. We have shown that carbohydrate ingestion facilitates creatine transport such that it reduces the variation between individuals.

Passwater: Can muscle creatine content be optimized by using lower doses?

Greenhaff: Yes, but it takes considerably longer. Lower-dose creatine supplementation (e.g., 3 grams a day for two weeks) is less effective in the short term at raising muscle creatine concentration than is a five-day regimen of 20 grams a day. **However, following four weeks of supplementation at this lower dose, muscle creatine accumulation is no different when regimens are compared**.

Passwater: Who discovered the creatine loading concept and when?

Greenhaff: Creatine loading came out of Dr. Eric Hultman's laboratory in the late 1980s, but his paper wasn't published until 1992. The results were so striking that the research had to be verified several times, looking at different doses. The idea of a loading phase and then a maintenance phase came out of my laboratory from 1993 through 1994, but in collaboration with Dr. Hultman. I want to make it clear that Dr. Hultman is the real pioneer in all of this work.

Dr. Greenhaff and his colleagues biopsied muscles to study the effect of creatine loading. They found that during creatine loading via the ingestion of 20 grams of creatine in solution each day for five days (four x 5-gram doses per day), which leads to an average increase in muscle creatine concentration of about 25 percent, approximately 30 percent is in the form of CP. The majority of muscle creatine retention occurs during the initial days of supplementation; e.g., about 30 percent of the administered dose is retained during the initial two days of supplementation, compared with 15 percent from days two to four. The natural time-course of muscle creatine decay following five days of 20 grams per day ingestion occurs over the course of several weeks rather than days. Earlier creatinine excretion studies showed that creatinine excretion doesn't increase immediately upon cessation of creatine supplementation and remains elevated for at least five weeks.

MAINTAINING THE CREATINE LOAD

It also appears that muscle creatine stores remain elevated for several weeks when the supplementation regimen of 20 grams per day for five days is followed by lower-dose supplementation (2 grams per day).

Researcher Anthony Almada relates that his experience suggests that serious competitors use a maintenance dose of 10 to 15 grams of creatine daily regardless of body weight. He notes that preliminary studies at the University of Nebraska suggest a higher maintenance dosage may increase the creatine response in terms of strength and body weight gain. Further studies are required to clarify this point.

The muscles do have an upper limit of creatine uptake and creatine storage, and taking more than 20 grams a day appears to offer no additional benefit. Several studies have shown that higher loading doses (up to 35 grams a day) do not promote greater muscle performance. However, the effects of higher doses upon body weight/composition have yet to be evaluated.

INCREASING CREATINE UPTAKE

Although the mechanisms involved in creatine uptake into muscles are not fully understood, it is believed that they include simple diffusion and perhaps active transport by the creatine transporter protein. Dr. Greenhaff and his colleagues have found that simple-sugar carbohydrates increase creatine uptake. Again, let's let Dr. Greenhaff tell us in his own words.

Passwater: You mentioned that carbohydrates can facilitate creatine transport into the muscle, and that this is a way in which poor responders can increase their efficiency of creatine loading. Do carbohydrates enhance total creatine-loading capacity?

Greenhaff: Yes, they do. The mechanism is not yet clear. Of course, it could be related to insulin availability because it's known that insulin has a number of functions, one of which is stimulation of membrane transport. So it could be via that mechanism but there are other ways. At the moment we don't really know, and that's something that needs to be answered from research.

The hormone insulin helps carbohydrates and amino acids pass through the membranes of cells. Insulin also can increase blood flow, which suggests that increases in insulin may deliver more creatine to muscle cells by providing more creatine-rich blood. Certain carbohydrates increase the amount of insulin in the blood, so at first it was thought that insulin was responsible for the increased uptake of creatine when it is consumed simultaneously with carbohydrates. However, a newer working hypothesis may be evolving which adds to the possible boosting effect of insulin.

When scientists added insulin to an in vitro laboratory system using animal-derived immature muscle cells to study creatine uptake, concentrations of insulin that would be encountered in daily physiological (real life) situations were found not to be potent enhancers of creatine uptake. However, very high concentrations of insulin, and the insulin mimic vanadate, boosted creatine retention. The isoflavone genistein, found in soy foods, was actually found to reduce cell creatine, which suggests that soy-rich diets may reduce muscle creatine retention. Vegetarians can display slightly lower muscle creatine content. These studies were published in 1996 by Dr. George Radda and his associates.

CREATINE TRANSPORTER

The mechanisms by which creatine can enter muscle cells are not fully understood at this time, but they are believed to include diffusion and transport by a transporter protein. It has been found that creatine uptake can be increased when hormones released during and after eating are present. This effect was at first associated with the hormone insulin, but insulin may be merely a marker of the events that lead to the release of other hormones. This will be discussed later under the topic of increasing creatine uptake.

When the diet provides large amounts of creatine for an extended period, a feedback mechanism is believed to send chemical messengers to the genetic material that regulates the production of this creatine transporter to shut down its production and reduce the number of available transporters. When dietary creatine is diminished again, the genetic material receives another chemical message to resume production of the transporter and increase the number of available transporters. The regulation of the genetic expression of this transporter is now under active research.

BUILDING MASSIVE MUSCLES

The goal then is to train by increasing the work that a muscle must do. This increased workload can be achieved in three ways:
- by increasing the force of contraction by using increased resistance such as lifting a heavier weight or pushing off or jumping with more explosive force
- by increasing the duration of time that the muscle is contracted
- by increasing the frequency of exercise

Creatine helps in all three ways:
- it helps build muscle mass which allows still greater force to be used
- it provides energy so that duration of exercise or work can be lengthened
- it speeds recovery so that exercise frequency can be increased

MUSCLE "CELL-VOLUMIZING" MAY FORCE MUSCLE GROWTH

Animal cell studies suggest that creatine may promote muscle growth by stimulating protein synthesis. There are two actions involved. The first is simply due to the increased work which muscle can produce due to the increased energy content of the muscle and the delay in muscle tiredness. The second way is a bonus that comes from the increased amount of creatine absorbed in the muscle tissue. As creatine is taken up into the muscle cells, it also associates with water. As more creatine is stored, more water may be brought into the muscle. This gives muscle a full or pumped feel and look, but it also may increase the volume of the muscle cells. When muscle cell volume is increased, it is thought that this triggers more protein and glycogen synthesis, reduces protein breakdown (proteolysis) and increases muscle mass. The muscle fibers become larger and stronger. This concept was coined "cell-volumizing" by researchers Anthony Almada and Ed Byrd.

For more information on the cell-volumizing phenomenon, I checked with Dr. Greenhaff to see just what we do know for sure scientifically, and how much is speculation at this time.

Passwater: Cell-volumizing or cell hydration-is that a real phenomenon or is this a myth?

Greenhaff: Scientifically speaking, I think people may be jumping the gun a little, taking information that has been gained from animal and muscle preparations and applying that directly to exercising humans. What is known is that if you increase the volume of a muscle cell in a laboratory situation, the changes in volume can have subsequent physiological responses. For example, it has been shown that an increase in cell volume can stimulate carbohydrate synthesis in muscle. But then to take that fact and apply it directly to human muscles and even take it a further step and say creatine has other effects because it potentially increases muscle water volume is really speculation. I think research in this area needs to be undertaken before we can make any more conclusive statements about it.

Passwater: So, this concept has not been fully verified by science at this time, but it does in fact have some basis based on preliminary animal studies.

Greenhaff: Yes.

SOME EVIDENCE THAT CREATINE IS A LACTIC ACID BUFFER IN INTERMITTENT EXERCISE

Another point that needs clarification is whether or not creatine is truly a lactic acid buffer. Early studies have suggested such a role, but later, better designed studies are equivocal. However, a new study by Dr. Michael Prevost of Louisiana State University confirms earlier studies by Dr. Hultman's group and adds important new information that indicates creatine may buffer lactic acid and improve recovery time in short-duration maximal-intensity exercise. The results are being reviewed by a major exercise physiology journal at this writing and will probably be published in the fall of 1997.

When muscles use the anaerobic energy system to contract during intense exercise, they produce lactic acid. Acids supply hydrogen ions which can interfere with muscle contraction, nerve conduction and energy production. Lactic acid build-up is partially responsible for that burning feeling that occurs as muscles become fatigued. This fatigue decreases with exercise frequency and duration. When one can't exercise any longer because the muscles burn and won't contract, it is probably due either to running out of energy or to excessive lactic acid build-up. Lactate (lactic acid without the "acid" [H^+] portion) concentration in the blood is a measure of the amount of lactic acid produced during exercise, which indicates the amount of anaerobic metabolism occurring.

A lactic acid buffer works by absorbing hydrogen ions (H^+) released during the energy producing reactions. Creatine absorbs hydrogen ions in the process of creatine phosphate transferring a high-energy phosphate group to ADP to form ATP:

$$CP + ADP + H^+ \rightleftharpoons ATP + C$$

The data are equivocal at this writing, but the biochemistry appears to be there. Thus, it is not only a possibility, but perhaps a probability that creatine can delay the onset of fatigue by reducing lactate build-up during very short bursts of exercise.

Even if creatine does not buffer lactic acid, creatine can extend the exercise or work period by virtue of increased energy stored in the muscles. In other words, you can train or perform longer because you have more muscle energy available.

Dr. Prevost points out that there are four important metabolic considerations that affect the performance of high-intensity intermittent exercise, the type of muscle function called upon in most sports:

- Maintenance of high energy phosphates (the phosphagen system)
- Recovery of high-energy phosphates during the brief rest periods
- Restoration of the ability to generate ATP during the exercise
- The management of adenine nucleotides (AMP, ADP, ATP)

Creatine supplementation can benefit all four stages. Before looking at Dr. Prevost's results, let's check with Dr. Paul Greenhaff about the concept that creatine reduces lactic acid build-up during prolonged exercise.

Passwater: Does creatine delay lactic acid build-up during exercise?

Greenhaff: Other groups are suggesting that yes, you can lower lactic acid production during exercise, and possibly you can during very, very short sprints or very, very short bouts of exercise-just a few seconds. But, in our hands, when exercise is sustained for more than five to six seconds, we see no effect on lactic acid production.

High-intensity, short-duration, intermittent exercise is what normally occurs in some sports. You go all out for five to ten seconds and then recover while coasting at a slower output until it's your turn again. You may run the ball and then recover in the huddle, or you may chase a fly ball and wait for the next batter or you may press a weight for several reps and then recover for the next set.

Dr. Prevost tested kinesiology students at LSU during bursts of maximal pedaling on a bike followed by brief recovery periods. Creatine's effect in delaying fatigue was particularly demonstrated in the tests where the subjects repeatedly pedaled at maximum speed for 10 seconds and rested for 20 seconds. In this 10/20 cycle of exercise, the placebo group would tire after about three minutes, but the creatine group never tired at all. The experiment was discontinued because the subjects who took creatine seemed as if they would be able to continue indefinitely at this rate.

Dr. Prevost's study is a confirmation of a study done by Dr. Eric Hultman's group, which studied very brief bouts (cycles) of cycling (on a bicycle ergometer) at two intensities. Creatine supplementation enhanced performance and the amount of exercise that could be completed at these high intensities, and also lowered blood lactate concentration and oxygen consumption. This study is discussed later in "The Scientific Studies" section as the Balsom 1993 Study.

Dr. Prevost is now with the Naval Operational Medicine

Institute in El Toro, California. I asked him to tell us about his research with creatine.

Passwater: Why did the creatine-supplemented group not tire during the 10/20 experiment?

Prevost: During short exercise bouts, a greater portion of the energy is supplied by the phosphagen system. This means that creatine loading can pack more creatine phosphate into the muscles to supply more ATP and to regenerate ATP quicker. Even a small amount of extra creatine phosphate significantly increases the relative amount of ATP resynthesized. This delays the need for energy from the glycolysis system, which is the producer of lactic acid.

Passwater: So there may be less lactate formed in the first place, rather than a diminishment of lactate that has formed from glycolysis. The net result is still less lactic acid build-up, so there is less fatigue. How about oxygen consumption?

Prevost: My studies also showed oxygen consumption was reduced by creatine supplementation. Since oxygen consumption is related to energy expenditure, we might conclude that exercise efficiency (work/cost) was also improved.

The details of Dr. Prevost's studies and other major studies are given in the section "The Scientific Studies."

Dr. Prevost's study involved short-duration, maximal-energy exercise. This involves the type of muscle use involved in sprinting, swinging a bat, chasing a fly ball, running a post pattern, or most any athletic or team event except long-distance running. In Dr. Prevost's studies, those taking creatine supplements outperformed those taking the placebo (inert look-alike supplement) at the point athletes would normally tire. Examples would include sprinters in the final heat after running qualifiers, an athlete competing in multiple events or backs running in the fourth quarter at the same speed as they can in the first quarter.

CREATINE CYCLING

The concept of "cycling" of sports supplements is a holdover from the use of steroid anabolic drugs. Cycling means to use the product for a while, then discontinue its use, and keep repeating this cycle of usage. Cycling was a necessity with steroid anabolic drugs because the drugs accumulated in the body and led to very severe adverse effects. By periodically discontinuing their use, the drug concentration stored in the body would decrease, hopefully below the levels causing adverse effects. There does not appear to be a need to cycle creatine in relation to safety and toxicity issues. However, even though there is no necessity to cycle creatine, the question should still be asked if cycling would produce additional benefit. Let's look at both what science can tell us and what user experience can tell us.

Dr. Paul Greenhaff comments about the effects of creatine supplementation as it pertains to the subject of creatine cycling.

Passwater: Does taking creatine supplements shut down endogenous creatine biosynthesis?

Greenhaff: Yes, in the amounts used for increased performance it does. So does eating large amounts of meat which, of course, contains creatine. It's a natural feedback mechanism. But what people should be clear about is that once creatine supplementation is stopped and the muscle levels then begin to decline, endogenous synthesis starts again. You have to remember that we are talking about people ingesting possibly 20 grams a day at least initially and dropping to lower maintenance doses of two or more grams per day. With normal diets, endogenous synthesis probably contributes one to two grams per day. So when you consume more than you normally would have to make, there is no need for the body to synthesize creatine.

Passwater: Does taking creatine supplements also reduce the creatine precursor, guanidine acetic acid (GAA) production?

Greenhaff: Essentially, GAA is needed only for creatine production, and if the body is getting all of the creatine it needs from the diet, then GAA production is also halted during the time of adequate creatine intake. GAA and creatine production both are activated again when dietary creatine decreases.

Passwater: Does creatine supplementation halt creatine transport?

Greenhaff: Well, initially it very much stimulates creatine transport. When the muscles are loaded with creatine, additional transport of creatine into the muscles does decline. This is merely a natural feedback mechanism resulting from the increase in muscle creatine content.

Passwater: Does creatine supplementation affect the production of creatine kinase, the enzyme needed to reconvert creatine back into creatine phosphate?

Greenhaff: I haven't seen any evidence to suggest that anywhere.

Passwater: Does creatine supplementation reduce the number of creatine receptor sites?

Greenhaff: There is no answer to that question. I don't believe that a creatine receptor site has ever been characterized. Researchers have identified a creatine transporter in muscle, but no one has measured the number of transporters and whether they change with creatine ingestion.

Sometimes experience teaches us a refinement or two beyond formal scientific studies. The above observations by Dr. Greenhaff may be your best bet. However, competitive athletes may wish to try the strategy suggested by researcher Anthony Almada. He points out that it is without scientific substantiation at this time, but based on what is known about creatine loading, this strategy may prove to enhance performance.

Almada suggests that two to three weeks before competition, athletes discontinue creatine supplementation and allow muscle creatine reserves to decline. It takes more than a month for the excess creatine to diffuse out of the muscle. Even if a longer time passes, the muscle creatine level will not dip below the previous base-line level. Even if muscle creatine returns to pre-supplementation level, few athletes experience a significant loss of strength or size during this type of creatine washout, suggesting that creatine supplementation contributes to a permanent ergogenic and anabolic effect in muscles. The urinary excretion of creatine will increase after about two to three days. Shortly thereafter, the creatine-transport protein synthesis should increase, along with an increase in the number of available transporters.

One week to ten days before competition, creatine loading may begin again, taken in combination with glucose or at least 16 ounces of orange juice or grape juice. Remember, the extra creatine loaded into the muscles has not yet had enough time to fully diffuse (empty). This time there should be enough creatine transport proteins to pack more creatine into the muscles while the muscles still contain more than a baseline amount of creatine already. The net result may be a renewed superloading of creatine.

THE SCIENTIFIC STUDIES

This book is based on the findings of many scientific studies. More than 50 pertinent to creatine metabolism and muscle physiology are listed in the bibliography. However, there are only eight key studies that form the basis for the proper use of creatine supplements to obtain optimal sports performance.

Harris 1992 Study

Let's begin with the seminal study by Dr. Eric Hultman's group, which is often referred to in writings about creatine as a 1992 study by Harris and colleagues. The research was actually done in Dr. Hultman's laboratory with his colleagues at the Karolinska Institute (Sweden) in the late 1980s, but it was not published in the scientific literature until 1992. The full reference is listed in the bibliography.

The importance of this study is that it showed that muscle creatine levels could be increased by 50 percent just by taking creatine supplements. This study helped set the parameters for creatine loading.

The study reported that supplementation with 5 grams of creatine monohydrate mixed into hot tea or coffee four or six times a day for two or more days resulted in a significant increase in the total creatine content of the quadriceps femoris muscle as measured in 17 volunteers. Those persons who initially had the lowest amount of creatine stored in the muscle had the biggest gains, which were in some cases up to 50 percent.

This study found that creatine uptake into muscle was the greatest during the first two days (32 percent). About 20 percent of the creatine increase was due to increased creatine phosphate content. There was no increase found in ATP stored in the resting muscle.

The study also found that when only one leg was exercised by pedaling the bicycle ergometer, it accumulated more creatine than the nonexercised leg. The average level of creatine before supplementation was 118 mmol/kg. The average after supplementation was 148.5 mmol/kg in the nonexercised leg and 162.2 mmol/kg in the exercised leg. Thus, the nonexercised leg increased its creatine store by about 25 percent and the exercised leg improved by 37 percent.

Greenhaff 1993 Study

This study is the first to show the benefits of creatine supplementation on intense exercise performance. The study is a collaboration involving Dr. Paul Greenhaff and colleagues with Dr. Eric Hultman and colleagues. The full reference is listed in the bibliography.

In this study, twelve volunteers undertook five bouts of 30 maximal voluntary isokinetic leg extension contractions, interspersed with one minute recovery periods, before and after five days of taking either a placebo or creatine supplement. The placebo was 6 grams of glucose per day and the creatine supplement was 5 grams of creatine (in the form of creatine monohydrate) plus 1 gram of glucose mixed into tea or coffee. Muscle torque production and blood lactate and ammonia levels were measured before and after exercise on each treatment.

There were no measurable differences in muscle peak torque production during exercise before and after taking the placebo. However, after taking the creatine supplement, muscle peak torque production was greater in all volunteers during the final ten contractions of exercise bout number one, throughout the entire range of exercise bout numbers two, three and four, and during contractions 11 - 20 of the final exercise bout number five, when compared with the corresponding measurements made before creatine supplementation.

The level of ammonia was lower during and after exercise in those supplemented with creatine, but no differences were found in blood lactate levels.

Balsom 1993 Study

This study by Dr. Eric Hultman's group showed that creatine supplementation decreased blood lactate, improved performance and increased muscle mass. The full reference is listed in the bibliography.

In this study, two intermittent high-intensity exercise regimens were performed before and after loading with either a placebo or a creatine monohydrate supplement (5 grams of creatine monohydrate plus 1 gram of glucose, five times daily for six days). Each exercise regimen consisted of ten six-second bouts of high-intensity cycling at two exercise intensities, 130 revolutions per minute (rpm) or 140 rpm, in a manner so that the same amount of exercise was performed before and after the administration period. The 140 rpm intensity was chosen to induce fatigue over the ten exercise bouts.

Sixteen male volunteers were randomly assigned to two experimental groups (placebo vs. creatine groups). There were no significant changes in any measured parameters in the placebo group. However, those receiving the creatine supplementation had enhanced performance towards the end of each exercise bout at 140 rpm, as measured by smaller declines in work output. Although the creatine-supplemented group performed more work, their blood lactate decreased from 10.8 to 9.1 mmol/liter and there was no change in oxygen uptake. The creatine group also demonstrated a body-weight gain of 2.4 pounds, with no significant change in the placebo group.

At the 130 rpm rate, the creatine-supplemented group also had 37 percent lower lactate build-up (7.0 vs 5.1), and the oxygen uptake was also lower. The researchers stated that the mechanisms responsible for the improved performance with creatine supplementation were probably due to both a higher initial muscle creatine phosphate availability and an increased rate of creatine phosphate resynthesis during recovery periods. The lower lactate accumulation may also be explained by these mechanisms.

Earnest 1995 Study

This is one of several studies in collaboration with Anthony Almada. It is the first study to show that creatine supplementation increased strength during weightlifting (bench press) and that the weight gain associated with creatine use was due to increases in muscle (lean body mass). These results were presented at the annual meeting of the American College of Sports Medicine in Indianapolis in May 1994 and at the National Strength and Conditioning Association (NSCA) National Conference in New Orleans in July 1994, later published in 1995. The complete reference is listed in the bibliography.

In this study, eight weight-trained men were randomly assigned to receive a placebo or creatine monohydrate supplement for 28 days. Prior to and immediately following the supplementation period, each volunteer was evaluated for body weight, body composition (via underwater weighing), and one repetition of the bench press at maximal weight. In addition, each volunteer also performed as many repetitions as possible at 70 percent of their pretest maximum bench press weight.

There were no changes in any measured parameter in the placebo group. In the creatine-supplemented group, the bench press maximum improved by 18 pounds (8.2 kilograms). The total amount of weight lifted as measured by the number of complete lifting repetitions (at the 70 percent maximum weight) times that weight improved by 971 pounds (441.3 kilograms). The number of repetitions at the 70 percent of maximum weight improved by four repetitions. An important new finding was that lean body weight increased by an average of 3.74 pounds (1.7 kilograms).

The same volunteers were also part of a study to determine if creatine monohydrate affected peak anaerobic power or anaerobic capacity. The volunteers performed three successive 30-second exercise tests called "Wingate tests," interspersed with five-minute recovery periods before and after two weeks of either placebo or creatine supplementation. The creatine supplementation consisted of taking 5 grams of creatine (from creatine monohydrate) plus 1 gram of glucose four times a day (daily total of 20 grams of creatine plus 4 grams of glucose).

The creatine supplementation produced significant increases in anaerobic capacity and decreased blood ammonia levels. The placebo group had no significant increase in anaerobic capacity and had higher blood ammonia levels. Neither group had a significant increase in peak anaerobic power. This was the first study to evaluate the effects of long-term (four-week) creatine supplementation. No adverse effects were reported by the volunteers, nor were there any adverse changes in blood chemistry.

Green 1996 Studies

Two studies were published by Dr. Paul Greenhaff's group in 1996 showing that ingesting simple carbohydrate (primarily glucose) in solution along with the creatine increased muscle creatine uptake, especially in those who responded poorly to straight creatine supplementation. Dr. Greenhaff discussed the possible mechanism involved earlier in this Guide in the section on creatine loading. The mechanism could involve insulin or other factors released during carbohydrate digestion and/or absorption. The references listed in the bibliography.

In the first of these two studies, four groups of volunteers received various combinations of creatine or placebo with or without added carbohydrate. Group A received creatine alone, Groups B and C received creatine plus a simple carbohydrate mixture and Group D received a placebo with no creatine or carbohydrate. Group C also exercised daily. The results indicate that the carbohydrate increased creatine retention and decreased creatine excretion. The exercise did not augment the creatine retention.

The second of these two studies involved two groups of volunteers, and muscle biopsies were also taken. There was a 60 percent improvement in muscle creatine retention in the group receiving both creatine and carbohydrate.

Kreider 1996 Study

In another study in collaboration with Almada, scientists from the University of Memphis, led by Dr. Richard B. Kreider, evaluated the effects on body composition during resistance training of supplementing with either a low-calorie creatine-containing mixture (also providing glutamine, taurine and yeast-RNA as active ingredients, and moderate quantities of protein and carbohydrate), a high-calorie protein/carbohydrate powder, or carbohydrate powder alone. The study was conducted for 28 days on 28 resistance-trained individuals.The complete reference is listed in the bibliography.

This study was the first to describe the body composition-modifying effects of a supplement containing creatine along with other compounds, and used a very sophisticated method (DEXA) to determine body composition. The researchers found a three-times greater increase in fat-free mass with the creatine mixture, compared to both the "protein plus carbohydrate" or "carbohydrate" supplements. Body fat mass did not increase in the creatine mixture or carbohydrate groups, but increased significantly in the high-calorie group. The researchers concluded that use of the creatine mixture"...resulted in a significantly greater increase in lean tissue weight, while fat weight was maintained."

In a follow-up study designed to duplicate the above findings, Dr. Kreider, Almada and colleagues tested the effects of five weeks of supplementation with either the same creatine mixture, or a similar mixture with a higher content of the active ingredients plus calcium alpha-ketoglutarate, or carbohydrate powder in university football players during an intensive off-season training period. After five weeks of supplementation, the two groups receiving the creatine mixtures gained significantly more fat-free weight than the carbohydrate group. Those taking the lower-dose creatine mixture gained 5.4 pounds of fat-free weight, while those taking the higher dose creatine mixture gained 7.6 pounds. These results were presented at the American College of Sports Medicine annual meeting in Minneapolis in Cincinnati in May of 1996, and have been submitted for publication. The full title of this abstract is listed in the bibliography.

Kreider 1997 Studies

In another double-blind study conducted by many of the same researchers, university football players receiving a creatine, glucose, taurine and electrolyte supplement displayed greater increases in strength and sprint capacity than players receiving the same supplement but without creatine. This study was presented at the American College of Sports Medicine annual meeting in May 1997, in Denver and the abstract was published in *Medicine and Science in*

Sports and Exercise (29 (5) Abstr. 833, 1997). Also, for the same group of athletes, those receiving the creatine-containing mixture gained twice as much fat-free mass as those receiving the mixture without creatine, with no changes in fat-mass in either group (*Med. Sci. Sports Ex.* 29 (5): Abstr. 832, 1997).

Prevost 1997 Study

This is the study by Dr. Mike Prevost discussed in the section in this guide on reducing blood lactate. The study was conducted at Louisiana State University in 1996. This study shows that creatine supplementation enhances exercise performance during very brief (less than ten seconds) high-intensity exercises that primarily stress the phosphagen system. Creatine may lead to a lower lactate accumulation because a creatine-loaded phosphagen system (creatine phosphate - ATP) can supply a larger amount of the energy needs during these bursts of exercise. Therefore, the muscle doesn't activate the glycolysis system as early and as aggressively; as a result, there is less blood lactate accumulation.

In this study, 18 volunteers from the LSU kinesiology department were divided into two groups, a placebo-control and, during the second phase of the study, a creatine-supplemented group. The creatine-supplemented group was also tested with placebos during the first phase of testing. This group was given creatine supplementation (18.5 grams of creatine monohydrate daily for five days followed by 10.3 grams daily for six days) before and during the second phase of testing. Both groups underwent identical testing protocols. Blood analyses and VO_2 measurements were taken during each test.

Dr. Prevost reports that creatine supplementation had a significant effect on time to exhaustion and thus total work output. The creatine-supplemented group showed a greater than 100 percent *increase* in time to exhaustion in phase 2 of the test, which involved repetitious cycles of 10-second pedaling at high-intensity followed by 20-second recovery periods. The placebo group showed no change.

Now here is the interesting part. The tests were halted at twice the performance time **because the volunteers on creatine reported "feeling very little fatigue and the ability to continue indefinitely."** Another variation of the test, in which the test cycle for each subject was to pedal for 20 seconds and recover for 40 seconds, also showed that creatine extended performance. Creatine increased the time to exhaustion by 62 percent.

Oxygen consumption increased with time, but the creatine-supplemented group showed a significantly lower oxygen-consumption rate than that of the placebo group during the 10/20 and 20/40 cycles. Blood lactate concentration increased with exercise time, but lactate concentration in the creatine- supplemented group was significantly lower than that in the placebo group in both the 10/20 and 20/40 cycles.

This study has been submitted to the *Research Quarterly For Sport and Exercise* and should be published during 1997.

CREATINE SUPPLEMENTS

If all of the protein one ate could be efficiently broken down into amino acids, and then all of the arginine, glycine and methionine so produced were efficiently converted into creatine, the body still would not produce more than approximately 2 grams of creatine, the amount needed daily to replace that lost in the urine. The same would be true if one merely took supplements of arginine, glycine and methionine. The best way to increase the amount of creatine in the muscles is to take creatine supplements along with a potent insulin-releasing carbohydrate such as glucose or sucrose and a small amount of sodium, an essential cofactor for creatine transport.

The most popular form of creatine in supplement form is creatine monohydrate. All of the published scientific studies have been conducted with creatine monohydrate. It is virtually tasteless and adequately soluble in water. Creatine monohydrate contains more creatine per weight of material than any other form. Creatine monohydrate is simply a molecule of creatine with a molecule of water attached. When creatine monohydrate dissolves in water, the molecule of water that was attached is released, as is the creatine. Creatine monohydrate thus contains 880 milligrams of "free" creatine in every gram of creatine monohydrate. In this form, creatine can be purified and stabilized.

Creatine phosphate (CP) is the form of creatine that drives the energy pump, but this is not the best form to use as a supplement to shuttle creatine into the muscles. None of the scientific studies have used creatine phosphate as the dietary source of creatine as it has never been shown to have an ergogenic or anabolic effect when taken orally. The goal is to get the creatine into muscles and then trap it there by converting it into creatine phosphate.

A molecule of creatine phosphate is actually one molecule of creatine bound to one phosphate group. A gram of creatine phosphate contains 623 milligrams of free creatine. Since the phosphate group weighs more than a molecule of water, a molecule of creatine phosphate weighs more than a molecule of creatine monohydrate. This means that a gram of creatine monohydrate contains 41 percent more creatine than a gram of creatine phosphate. Creatine phosphate is also very expensive.

Creatine citrate is more soluble than creatine monohydrate, but creatine citrate is a less concentrated form. Creatine citrate contains approximately 400 milligrams of free creatine in every gram of creatine citrate. In a glass, creatine citrate may be more soluble than creatine monohydrate, but keep in mind that creatine monohydrate contains more than twice the free creatine. Dr. Paul Greenhaff has shared unpublished data with me showing that there appears to be no difference between the two forms in terms of whole-body creatine retention. Creatine citrate is not as palatable as creatine monohydrate and it is more expensive. None of the published scientific studies has used creatine citrate as a dietary source of creatine.

CREATINE PARTNERS

Combining creatine (plus carbohydrate) with good-quality protein and/or the amino acids prevalent in muscle protein is a good idea. These amino acids include glutamine, branched-chain amino acids (valine, leucine and isoleucine) and taurine.

Studies suggest that glutamine helps regulate protein synthesis in skeletal muscle and may help protect muscle tissue from being degraded (catabolism). The body needs glutamine for many reasons, especially during physical stress such as exercise. When other regions of the body run low in glutamine, the reserves stored in muscles are called upon. When glutamine is released from muscles, some degradation of muscle tissue may occur. The strategy of providing glutamine during exercise is to provide these other regions of the body with a dietary source of glutamine rather than having the glutamine stores of muscles depleted. There is some suggestion that glutamine, under certain conditions, may contribute to cell volumization, but the scientific evidence of such an effect is very weak at this time.

Taurine has been reported to be the second most abundant free amino acid present in human skeletal muscle. Taurine is not involved in muscle fiber structure, but is prevalent in type I muscle fibers attached to magnesium ions. Magnesium is important to ATP because it stabilizes the position of the phosphate groups in ATP. Animal studies suggest that taurine may also potentiate the action of insulin. As with glutamine, there is a weak suggestion that taurine may be anti-catabolic and cell-volumizing.

Water is critical to the performance enhancement of creatine. Dr. Greenhaff has emphasized the importance of administering creatine in solution. Usually, powders are used, but tablets can be used if adequate water is consumed simultaneously. The water is taken into the muscle cells to promote cell volumization. This is not the same as water retention. Water retention produces bloating and smooths the appearances of muscles, similar to having an extra layer of fat. In the case of creatine, water is drawn into the muscle and bound with the creatine phosphate. This produces a very noticeable hardened and pumped effect.

SAFETY

The good news about creatine is that it is safe, even when taken in the quantities used by athletes. There have been no adverse effects reported in any of the studies other than the usual gastric upset or intolerance that any compound is known to cause in a few people. Although safety studies have not been conducted with people taking large amounts of creatine over many years, there are no suggestions or mechanisms known that would suggest to researchers that long-term studies would show anything different.

One study conducted with a group of men and women 32 to 70 years of age found that creatine loading at 20 grams per day for five days, followed by a 10-gram maintenance dose for 51 days, produced no adverse effects. However, this regimen did produce some very important benefits other than performance enhancement. **There was a 22 percent decrease in VLDL-cholesterol and a 23 percent decrease in blood triglyceride level.** Both VLDL-cholesterol and triglycerides are complementary risk factors in heart disease and adult-onset diabetes. The study also found a decrease in the concentration of blood sugar after an overnight fast, suggesting that creatine may improve the action of insulin. Earlier studies point to creatine reducing blood sugar in diabetic individuals.

As discussed earlier, there is no need to cycle creatine. However, I asked Dr. Greenhaff to discuss some of the other concerns raised by athletes.

Passwater: Does creatine supplementation increase creatine excretion?

Greenhaff: Yes, it does increase creatine excretion by virtue of the fact that once you have saturated muscle-creatine uptake, then the body just naturally excretes any creatine that is available in plasma, in circulation. It's just a natural mechanism.

Passwater: Does taking creatine supplements increase thirst?

Greenhaff: To be blunt, I don't know. The most effective way to take creatine is in solution, so you already are in fact taking fluids in that way. We haven't seen any individuals who have mentioned they have increased thirst. Certainly, in a situation where you are trying to optimize creatine transport, you are ingesting further fluids in the form of carbohydrate solution. If you are taking creatine supplements in solution form as our research suggests is the most efficient way, there should be no increase in thirst.

Passwater: Does increased creatine spill into the urine increase the volume of urine?

Greenhaff: No, what we have actually found is during the initial days of supplementation you actually get a decrease in urinary volume, but then after two days your urinary volume returns to normal. That's when you are ingesting creatine monohydrate on its own. If you are ingesting a solution of carbohydrates in conjunction with the creatine, then your urinary volume actually increases just because that you are ingesting more fluids.

LEGALITY

Creatine is not a steroid or drug. It is made in our bodies and is normally present in the diet. It is safe, legal and allowable for competition. It has not been banned by any sports association or government agency. Since it is present in everyone's blood and everyone excretes some creatine in the urine, there would be no practical way to test for creatine supplementation if it were to be banned.

BIBLIOGRAPHY

Almada, A., Mitchell, T., and Earnest, C. (1996). Impact of chronic creatine supplementation on serum enzyme concentrations. *FASEB J* 10(3):4567.

Arnold, D. L., Matthews, P. M., & Radda, G. K. (1984). Metabolic recovery after exercise and the assessment of mitochondrial function in vivo in human skeletal muscle by means of 31P NMR. *Magn Reson Med*, 1(3), 307-315.

Balsom, P. D., Ekblom, B., Soderlund, K., Sjodin, B., and Hultman, E. (1993) Creatine supplementation and dynamic high-intensity intermittent exercise. *Scand. J. Med. Sci. Sports.* 3:143-149.

Balsom, P. D., Soderlund, K., & Ekblom, B. (1994). Creatine in humans with special reference to creatine supplementation. *Sports Med*, 18(4), 268-280.

Balsom, P. D., Soderlund, K., Sjodin, B., & Ekblom, B. (1995). Skeletal muscle metabolism during short duration high-intensity exercise: influence of creatine supplementation. *Acta Physiol Scand*, 154(3), 303-310.

Birch, R., Noble, D., & Greenhaff, P. L. (1994). The influence of dietary creatine supplementation on performance during repeated bouts of maximal isokinetic cycling in man. *Eur J Appl Physiol*, 69(3), 268-276.

Boehm, E. A., Radda, G. K., Tomlin, H., & Clark, J. F. (1996). The utilisation of creatine and its analogues by cytosolic and mitochondrial creatine kinase. *Biochim Biophys Acta*, 1274(3), 119-128.

Buysse, A. M., Delanghe, J. R., De Buyzere, M. L., De Scheerder, I. K., De Mol, A. M., & Noens, L. (1990). Enzymatic erythrocyte creatine determinations as an index for cell age. *Clin Chim Acta*, 187(2), 155-162.

Byrnes, W. C., Clarkson, P. M., White, J. S., Hsieh, S. S., Frykman, P. N., & Maughan, R. J. (1985). Delayed onset muscle soreness following repeated bouts of downhill running. *J Appl Physiol*, 59(3), 710-715.

Casey, A., Constantin-Teodosiu, D., Howell, S., Hultman, E., & Greenhaff, P. L. (1996). Creatine ingestion favorably affects performance and muscle metabolism during maximal exercise in humans. *Am J Physiol*, 271(1 Pt 1), E31-7.

Clark, J. F., Kemp, G. J., & Radda, G. K. (1995). The creatine kinase equilibrium, free [ADP] and myosin ATPase in vascular smooth muscle cross-bridges. *J Theor Biol*, 173(2), 207-211.

Cooke, W. H., Grandjean, P. W., & Barnes, W. S. (1995). Effect of oral creatine supplementation on power output and fatigue during bicycle ergometry. *J Appl Physiol*, 78(2), 670-673.

Delanghe, J., De Slypere, J. P., De Buyzere, M., Robbrecht, J., Wieme, R., & Vermeulen, A. (1989). Normal reference values for creatine, creatinine, and carnitine are lower in vegetarians [letter]. *Clin Chem*, 35(8), 1802-1803.

Duthie, G. G., Robertson, J. D., Maughan, R. J., & Morrice, P. C. (1990). Blood antioxidant status and erythrocyte lipid peroxidation following distance running. *Arch Biochem Biophys*, 282(1), 78-83.

Earnest, C. P., Snell, P. G., Rodriguez, R., Almada, A. L., & Mitchell, T. L. (1995). The effect of creatine monohydrate ingestion on anaerobic power indices, muscular strength and body composition. *Acta Physiol Scand*, 153(2), 207-209.

Earnest, C. P., Almada, A. L., & Mitchell, T. L. (1996). High-performance capillary electrophoresis-pure creatine monohydrate reduces blood lipids in men and women. *Clin Sci (Colch)*, 91(1), 113-118.

Field, M. L., Unitt, J. F., Radda, G. K., Henderson, C., & Seymour, A. M. (1991). Age-dependent changes in cardiac muscle metabolism upon replacement of creatine by beta- guanidinopropionic acid. *Biochem Soc Trans*, 19(2), 208S

Field, M. L., Clark, J. F., Henderson, C., Seymour, A. M., & Radda, G. K. (1994). Alterations in the myocardial creatine kinase system during chronic anaemic hypoxia. *Cardiovasc Res*, 28(1), 86-91.

Fitch, C. D., & Chevli, R. (1980). Inhibition of creatine and phosphocreatine accumulation in skeletal muscle and heart. *Metabolism*, 29(7), 686-690.

Forrester, W., Maughan, R. J., Broom, J., & Whiting, P. H. (1996). Muscle protein release following down hill walking. *Biochem Soc Trans*, 24(2), 318S

Gordon, A., Hultman, E., Kaijser, L., Kristjansson, S., Rolf, C. J., Nyquist, O., & Sylven, C. (1995). Creatine supplementation in chronic heart failure increases skeletal muscle creatine phosphate and muscle performance. *Cardiovasc Res*, 30(3), 413-418.

Green, A. L., Hultman, E., Macdonald, I. A., Sewell, D. A., & Greenhaff, P. L. (1996). Carbohydrate ingestion augments skeletal muscle creatine accumulation during creatine supplementation in humans. *Am J Physiol*, 271(5 Pt 1), E821-6.

Green, A. L., Simpson, E. J., Littlewood, J. J., MacDonald, I. A., & Greenhaff, P. L. (1996) Carbohydrate ingestion augments creatine retention during creatine feeding in humans. *Acta Physiol Scand*, 158:195-202.

Greenhaff, P. L., Casey, A., Short, A. H., Harris, R., Soderlund, K., & Hultman, E. (1993). Influence of oral creatine supplementation of muscle torque during repeated bouts of maximal voluntary exercise in man. *Clin Sci (Colch)*, 84(5), 565-571.

Greenhaff, P. L., Bodin, K., Soderlund, K., & Hultman, E. (1994). Effect of oral creatine supplementation on skeletal muscle phosphocreatine resynthesis. *Am J Physiol*, 266(5 Pt 1), E725-30.

Greenhaff, P. L. (1995). Creatine and its application as an ergogenic aid. *Int J Sport Nutr*, 5 Suppl, S100-10.

Harris, R. C., Hultman, E., & Nordesjo, L. O. (1974). Glycogen, glycolytic intermediates and high-energy phosphates determined in biopsy samples of musculus quadriceps femoris of man at rest. Methods and variance of values. *Scand J Clin Lab Invest*, 33(2), 109-120.

Harris, R. C., Soderlund, K., & Hultman, E. (1992). Elevation of creatine in resting and exercised muscle of normal subjects by creatine supplementation. *Clin Sci (Colch)*, 83(3), 367-374.

Hellsten-Westing, Y., Norman, B., Balsom, P. D., & Sjodin, B. (1993). Decreased resting levels of adenine nucleotides in human skeletal muscle after high-intensity training. *J Appl Physiol*, 74(5), 2523-2528.

Hultman, E., Soderlund, K., Timmons, J. A., Cederblad, G., & Greenhaff, P. L. (1996). Muscle creatine loading in men. *J Appl Physiol*, 81(1), 232-237.

Kemp, G. J., Taylor, D. J., Radda, G. K., & Rajagopalan, B. (1992). Bio-energetic changes in human gastrocnemius muscle 1-2 days after strenuous exercise. *Acta Physiol Scand*, 146(1), 11-14.

Kemp, G. J., & Radda, G. K. (1993a). Control of intracellular concentrations of 'bioenergetic' metabolites in skeletal muscle. *Biochem Soc Trans*, 21(2), 177S

Kemp, G. J., Taylor, D. J., & Radda, G. K. (1993b). Control of phosphocreatine resynthesis during recovery from exercise in human skeletal muscle. *NMR Biomed*, 6(1), 66-72.

Korge, P. (1995a). Factors limiting adenosine triphosphatase function during high intensity exercise. Thermodynamic and regulatory considerations. *Sports Med*, 20(4), 215-225.

Korge, P., & Campbell, K. B. (1995b). The importance of ATPase microenvironment in muscle fatigue: a hypothesis. *Int J Sports Med*, 16(3), 172-179.

Kreider, R., Grindstaff, P., Wood, L., Bullen, D., Klesges, R., Lotz, D., Davis, M., Cantler, E.,& Almada, A. Effects of ingesting a lean mass-promoting supplement during resistance training on isokinetic performance. *Medicine and Science in Sports and Exercise*, 28(5): Abstr. 214 (1996).

Kreider, R. B., Klesges, R., Harmon, K., Grindstaff, P., Ramsey, L., Bullen, D., Wood, L., Li, Y., & Almada, A. (1996). Effects of ingesting supplements designed to promote lean tissue accretion on body composition during resistance training. *Int J Sport Nutr*, 6(3), 234-246.

Lindinger, M. I., Heigenhauser, G. J., & Spriet, L. L. (1987). Effects of intense swimming and tetanic electrical stimulation on skeletal muscle ions and metabolites. *J Appl Physiol*, 63(6), 2331-2339.

Maughan, R. J. (1995). Creatine supplementation and exercise performance. *Int J Sport Nutr*, 5(2), 94-101.

McCann, D. J., Mole, P. A., & Caton, J. R. (1995). Phosphocreatine kinetics in humans during exercise and recovery. *Med Sci Sports Exerc, 27*(3), 378-389.

Radda, G. K., Odoom, J., Kemp, G., Taylor, D. J., Thompson, C., & Styles, P. (1995). Assessment of mitochondrial function and control in normal and diseased states. *Biochim Biophys Acta, 1271*(1), 15-19.

Radda, G. K. (1996). Control of energy metabolism during muscle contraction. *Diabetes, 45* Suppl 1, S88-92.

Redondo, D. R., Dowling, E. A., Graham, B. L., Almada, A. L., & Williams, M. H. (1996). The effect of oral creatine monohydrate supplementation on running velocity. *Int J Sport Nutr, 6*(3), 213-221.

Robertson, J. D., Maughan, R. J., & Davidson, R. J. (1988). Changes in red cell density and related indices in response to distance running. *Eur J Appl Physiol, 57*(2), 264-269.

Robertson, J. D., Maughan, R. J., Duthie, G. G., & Morrice, P. C. (1991). Increased blood antioxidant systems of runners in response to training load [see comments]. *Clin Sci (Colch), 80*(6), 611-618.

Sahlin, K., Harris, R. C., & Hultman, E. (1975). Creatine kinase equilibrium and lactate content compared with muscle pH in tissue samples obtained after isometric exercise. *Biochem J, 152*(2), 173-180.

Sahlin, K., Harris, R. C., & Hultman, E. (1979). Resynthesis of creatine phosphate in human muscle after exercise in relation to intramuscular pH and availability of oxygen. *Scand J Clin Lab Invest, 39*(6), 551-558.

Shoubridge, E. A., Jeffry, F. M., Keogh, J. M., Radda, G. K., & Seymour, A. M. (1985b). Creatine kinase kinetics, ATP turnover, and cardiac performance in hearts depleted of creatine with the substrate analogue beta-guanidinopropionic acid. *Biochim Biophys Acta, 847*(1), 25-32.

Sipila, I., Rapola, J., Simell, O., & Vannas, A. (1981). Supplementary creatine as a treatment for gyrate atrophy of the choroid and retina. *N Engl J Med, 304*(15), 867-870.

Soderlund, K., & Hultman, E. (1990). ATP content in single fibres from human skeletal muscle after electrical stimulation and during recovery. *Acta Physiol Scand, 139*(3), 459-466.

Spincemaille, J., Delanghe, J., De Buyzere, M., Breemeersch, M., & Blaton, V. (1984). Evaluation of three current methods for the determination of creatine kinase-MB catalytic activity. *J Clin Chem Clin Biochem, 22*(9), 603-607.

Spriet, L. L., Lindinger, M. I., Heigenhauser, G. J., & Jones, N. L. (1986). Effects of alkalosis on skeletal muscle metabolism and performance during exercise. *Am J Physiol, 251*(5 Pt 2), R833-9.

Stroud, M. A., Holliman, D., Bell, D., Green, A. L., Macdonald, I. A., & Greenhaff, P. L. (1994). Effect of oral creatine supplementation on respiratory gas exchange and blood lactate accumulation during steady-state incremental treadmill exercise and recovery in man. *Clin Sci (Colch), 87*(6), 707-710.

Unitt, J. F., Radda, G. K., & Seymour, A. M. (1993). The acute effects of the creatine analogue, beta-guanidinopropionic acid, on cardiac energy metabolism and function. *Biochim Biophys Acta, 1143*(1), 91-96.

Vandenberghe, K., Gillis, N., Van Leemputte, M., Van Hecke, P., Vanstaple, F., & Hespel, P. (1996). Caeffeine counteracts the ergogenic action of muscle creatine loading. *J Appl Physiol, 80*(2):452-457.

Walker, J. B. (1979). Creatine : biosynthesis, regulation, and function. *Adv Enzymol Relat Areas Mol Biol, 50*, 177-242.

Wibom, R., Soderlund, K., Lundin, A., & Hultman, E. (1991). A luminometric method for the determination of ATP and phosphocreatine in single human skeletal muscle fibres. *J Biolumin Chemilumin, 6*(2), 123-129.

Woznicki, D. T., & Walker, J. B. (1980). Utilization of cyclocreatine phosphate, and analogue of creatine phosphate, by mouse brain during ischemia and its sparing action on brain energy reserves. *J Neurochem, 34*(5), 1247-1253.

GLOSSARY

adenosine diphosphate	ADP, a compound that stores energy, but less than ATP
adenosine monophosphate	AMP, a compound that stores energy, but less than ADP or ATP
adenosine nucleotides	AMP, ADP and ATP
adenosine triphosphate	ATP, a compound that stores more energy than AMP or ADP
acetyl CoA	acetyl coenzyme A, a critical two-carbon compound that is involved in the intermediate step between anaerobic glycosis and the Krebs cycle
actin	a protein in muscle fibers that acts with myosin to bring about contraction and relaxation
ADP	adenosine diphosphate
aerobic	processes dependent on oxygen
AMP	adenosine monophosphate
anabolism	the process of building larger compounds and cellular matter from simpler compounds-such as in the building of muscle fiber from nutrients
anaerobic	process independent of oxygen
ATP	adenosine triphosphate
ATP-energy	the energy contained in ATP
catabolism	the destruction of complex components into smaller components-such as the breakdown of muscle tissue or the release of energy from ATP
DEXA	dual energy x-ray absorptiometry, a method of scanning the body to measure bone, fat, and fat-free/soft tissue mass
electron	a negatively charged elementary particle that has a specific charge, mass and spin. Electrons orbit the nucleus of an atom
endogenous	originating within the body
ergogenic	work-producing
ergometer	a device to measure the amount of work performed
glucose	a simple sugar that provides ready fuel to produce energy
glycogen	a simple polysaccharide that is a fuel source that can be stored in the muscles. It is readily broken down to produce glucose
glycosis	the breaking down of glycogen to produce glucose
gyrate atrophy	a muscle wasting disease in which the atrophy worsens in a downward spiral

half-life	the time required to reduce the level of a compound to one half of its initial value
HMB	beta-hydroxy-beta-methylbutyrate, a dietary supplement that helps build muscle mass, strength and health
in vitro	done in chemical glassware outside of the body
in vivo	done in living bodies
isokinetic	a form of exercise in which maximal force is exerted by a muscle at each point throughout the range of motion as the muscle contracts
kinesiology	the scientific study of muscle activity, and of the anatomy, physiology, and the mechanics of movement of body parts
Krebs cycle	also called "citric acid cycle"-a sequence of enzymatic reactions involving the metabolism of carbon chains of sugars, fatty acids, and amino acids to produce high-energy phosphate bonds, carbon dioxide and water
mitochondrion	a small organelle within the cytoplasm of a cell that produces energy
muscle torque	a muscle force causing rotation or torsion
myosin	a protein that makes up about one-half of the proteins in muscle fibers
nuclei	the plural of nucleus
nucleus	the central controlling body within a cell, also the center of an atom
orbital	the path that an electron takes circumnavigating the nucleus of an atom
phosphagen system	the creatine-based system that produces immediate energy for muscle movement. This is also called the direct phosphorylation system or ATP-CP system
type I muscle fiber	red, slow twitch muscle fibers
type II muscle fiber	white, fast-twitch muscle fibers
urea	a compound that functions to remove ammonia from the body via urine. The catabolism of proteins releases ammonia. A molecule of urea combines two molecules of ammonia with an atom of carbon and an atom of oxygen
URL	Uniform (also called Universal) Resource Locator, the name of addresses on the Inetrnet
VO_2	the symbol for oxygen uptake